Katrine Stenlund

Intensive care

Katrine Stenlund

Intensive care

The significance of gender

LAP LAMBERT Academic Publishing

Impressum / Imprint

Bibliografische Information der Deutschen Nationalbibliothek: Die Deutsche Nationalbibliothek verzeichnet diese Publikation in der Deutschen Nationalbibliografie; detaillierte bibliografische Daten sind im Internet über http://dnb.d-nb.de abrufbar.
Alle in diesem Buch genannten Marken und Produktnamen unterliegen warenzeichen-, marken- oder patentrechtlichem Schutz bzw. sind Warenzeichen oder eingetragene Warenzeichen der jeweiligen Inhaber. Die Wiedergabe von Marken, Produktnamen, Gebrauchsnamen, Handelsnamen, Warenbezeichnungen u.s.w. in diesem Werk berechtigt auch ohne besondere Kennzeichnung nicht zu der Annahme, dass solche Namen im Sinne der Warenzeichen- und Markenschutzgesetzgebung als frei zu betrachten wären und daher von jedermann benutzt werden dürften.

Bibliographic information published by the Deutsche Nationalbibliothek: The Deutsche Nationalbibliothek lists this publication in the Deutsche Nationalbibliografie; detailed bibliographic data are available in the Internet at http://dnb.d-nb.de.
Any brand names and product names mentioned in this book are subject to trademark, brand or patent protection and are trademarks or registered trademarks of their respective holders. The use of brand names, product names, common names, trade names, product descriptions etc. even without a particular marking in this work is in no way to be construed to mean that such names may be regarded as unrestricted in respect of trademark and brand protection legislation and could thus be used by anyone.

Coverbild / Cover image: www.ingimage.com

Verlag / Publisher:
LAP LAMBERT Academic Publishing
ist ein Imprint der / is a trademark of
OmniScriptum GmbH & Co. KG
Heinrich-Böcking-Str. 6-8, 66121 Saarbrücken, Deutschland / Germany
Email: info@lap-publishing.com

Herstellung: siehe letzte Seite /
Printed at: see last page
ISBN: 978-3-659-64286-9

Copyright © 2014 OmniScriptum GmbH & Co. KG
Alle Rechte vorbehalten. / All rights reserved. Saarbrücken 2014

TABLE OF CONTENTS

INTRODUCTION — 5

BACKGROUND — 6

The country Jordan — 6

Intensive care — 7
Care in intensive care — 8

Gender perspective — 9
Sex differences in health care — 11
Sex differences in intensive care — 12

RATIONALE OF THE PROBLEM — 13

AIM — 13

METHOD — 13

Choice of method — 13
Quantitative approach — 15
Qualitative approach — 15

Gain access — 15
Study criteria — 16
Description of the intensive care units — 17
Pilot study — 19

Accomplish the observations — 20

Analyze collected data — 21

Ethical considerations — 23

RESULT — 24

Work within the intensive care area — 24
Family — 24
Cooperation — 25
Environment — 25

Observations in time and activity — 26
Time distribution — 27
Performed activities — 28

DISCUSSION	*30*
Discussion of the method	*30*
Observation schedule	30
Field notes	31
Access	32
Performance	33
Discussion of the result	*35*
Communication	35
Priority according to interest	36
Severity in illness	37
Differences in organization	38
Quantity or quality	38
Practical implications	39
CONCLUSION	*39*
ACKNOWLEDGEMENTS	*39*
REFERENCES	*40*
Appendix 1	*45*
Agreement in English from Jordan University Hospital	45
Agreement in Arabic from Jordan University Hospital	46
Appendix 2	*48*
Observation schedule	48
Elucidation of the activities	49
Appendix 3	*50*
Information letter to the nurses	50
Appendix 4	*51*
Result of the thematic content analyze	51

INTRODUCTION

This thesis is a result of a scholarship called Minor Field Study (MFS). The scholarship is founded by Sida; the Swedish International Development Cooperation Agency, which is a government agency under the Ministry for Foreign Affairs. Sida's general goal is to contribute to create a possibility for poor people to improve their living conditions (Sida, 2008). Their specific goal of MFS is to give students in Swedish universities and colleges an opportunity to acquire knowledge about development issues and to foster internationalization. The scholarship is supposed to encourage students to gather their material for a bachelor or master degree thesis or project in a developing country (Sida, 2009). To find out which countries counts as developing, the Development Assistance Committee defines a list of the present countries which the scholarship is provided for (Programkontoret, 2009).

When I found out about this opportunity; that I through my exam work, can study something that can contribute to a more professional intensive care in a developing country, I knew I wanted to apply. The choice of country for my thesis fell on Jordan since I find it interesting to see a country that in many ways are very different from my own. Compared to Sweden, Jordan has a strong religious culture and a history of many wars and different conquerors which has given it a unique mix of people. In some areas Jordan is still considered a developing country and in some areas, for example within the healthcare, it is world leading (Landguiden, 2009).

I have before this scholarship been both travelling and working abroad, which has made me observant on how varying expectations people from different cultures have on the medical care. I have also learned how important it is to be able to meet a patient or a relative from their point of view and be able to talk to them in terms they understand. Many of the foreign people, who today live in Sweden, come from the Middle East and I have met and will continue to meet them in my profession as a nurse. So I hope I will not only add to develop Jordan's intensive care, I also hope to develop my own understanding. Sharing my new views of intensive care with colleges in Sweden, I hope I will also add to develop the Swedish intensive care.

BACKGROUND

The country Jordan

The Hashemite Kingdom of Jordan, in daily talk called Jordan, is a monarchy in the Middle East in Asia (Landguiden, 2009). It border on Syria in the north, Iraq in east, Saudi Arabia in east and south and State of Palestine in west (Jordan, 2009:A). Arabic is the mainly spoken language but English is understood above all in the cities as a result of British influence during 1916-1946 and since English is taught in school. In 1946 Jordan won independence after having been ruled by a many different masters during the years. As a result of that and of the fact that Jordan, since the independence, has received a lot of refugees from the surrounding countries, the community is colored by numerous cultures (Fisher, 1996). The Palestinians represent with its 60% the largest group (Nationalencyklopedin, 2009:A) of Jordan's 5,9 million inhabitants (Department of Statistics, 2009). Most of the people live in towns of which the capital Amman is the largest with approximately 2,3 million citizens (Department of Statistics, 2008). The population is young and the median age is 20,3 years. A majority of the employees work within the public administration or wholesale and retail trade. 10,3% of the male population and 25,6% of the female population is unemployed. (Department of Statistics, 2007). Connell (1987) argue that men are more likely than women to get a paid employment but that women work just as much but preferable within non paid areas such as agriculture, household duties and taking care of and raise the children. This is supported by the fact that one of the traditional believes of Islam is that the male and the female have different tasks in the family. The female is supposed to take care of the home and raise the children while the male is supposed to work and provide for the family. The male is also the head of the family and he is the one who will make the big decisions and be the guardian for his wife and daughter (Heine, 2006). Even under these conditions over one third of the Jordanians chose to work abroad to be able to earn money to send home. The country is dependent on foreign aid and development loans but the tourism is improving thanks to the ancient cities of Petra and Jerash and the proximity to many biblical sites (Fisher).

Jordan's official religion is Islam and over 80% of the inhabitants belong to the branch called Sunni Muslims. This does not automatically make Jordan an Islamic state but the religion play an important role in many areas in the society and for the identity of people (Nationalencyklopedin, 2009:B). The king, Abdullah II, descends in an unbroken line from the Prophet Muhammad and in his official position he is in charge of almost every decision regarding the country and he is immune of any liability and responsibility. The constitution of Jordan was approved in 1952 and tells that power belongs to the people. There shall be no discrimination between Jordanians on account of race, religion or language. Work, education and equal opportunities shall be given to all as far as possible, why elementary education is free and compulsory and merits are the only thing which counts to get a work. The constitution also guarantees freedom of the individual, his dwelling and property (King Abdullah II, 2008). Press and opinions are free except under martial law but the Arab Archives Institute declares that the government holds majority of the shares in the newspapers and does not tolerate open criticism of the ruling (International Press Institute, 2007). Since 1989 a number of reforms have been implemented to increase the liberty, stability and modernity and the country is guided towards democratization (Jordan, 2009:B).

Intensive care

Jordan has a good health care standard, in some fields the techniques are world leading. A health care system is developed which guarantee free care and there are many different hospitals to choose from; private, governmental, military, charity and university hospitals (Landguiden, 2009). There are 11029 beds for patients allocated to 103 hospitals throughout the country (Department of Statistics, 2007). Jordan University Hospital is the first of now two existing university hospitals in the country. It was established as hospital in 1973, became a university hospital in 1975 and has a capacity of 540 beds (UJ Hospital, 2009). In one year around more than 400 000 patients are treated in inpatient wards, almost 300 000 in the outpatient clinics and almost 300 000 patients are admitted as emergency cases (UJ Hospital, 2006). The intensive care is divided into seven units: pediatric, medical, surgical 1, surgical 2, neurologic, cardiac and coronary intervention care.

The definition of intensive care is the same as for critical care; *"the specialized care of patients whose conditions are life-threatening and who require comprehensive care and constant monitoring, usually in intensive care units"* (Medicine Net, 2009). Larsson and Rubertsson (2005) wrote that the work usually is both physical and psychological demanding in a stressful surrounding. In the same time as it is important that things are detected and carried out fast, the personnel has a big responsibility to handle and talk to intensive care patients and their relatives and to coordinate their work with the others in the caring team around each intensive care patient. Since the personnel meet critical situations almost each workday it is important they get opportunities to talk and reflect over their work and feelings.

The intensive care patients' wide range conditions and the high-technological setting demand personnel who have an extensive education and competence. In Jordan, a four year long program in Bachelor of Science in Nursing, has to be completed before practicing intensive care as a nurse. The goal is that at least the unit's supervisor and the nurse in charge should have completed an additional two year long Master program in Clinical Critical Nursing. To be accepted to one of these programs very good grades are needed, at least 90% of the grades have to be of the highest value. Many of the nurses with a Master's degree, after graduation chose to work as instructors at universities or as nurses abroad and do not continue to work at the units, why the mentioned goal is tough to achieve (J. O. Halabi, personal communication, April 30, 2009).

Care in intensive care

Autonomy is one essential right for every person within the health care system. It means that a patient has the right to make own decisions in every situation. If the patient is unable to express his/her own wishes, their wishes and values expressed through for example relatives, shall be respected and accepted. Autonomy also means that every person who is affected by a decision shall have the possibility to influence the decision. This clearly shows that especially the patient but also the relatives and the personnel, have the right to take a part in the decision making within the intensive care. That is one of four principles whose aim is to provide a care as equal as possible for everybody. The second principle is justice which purpose is to provide an equal care to everyone, regardless of money, age, race, religion and sex. Together with the last two principles; do good and not hurt, they form a strategy to give each patient the most optimum care possible but also the right to say no to treatment (Larsson & Rubertsson, 2005).

During an intensive care stay this is often more problematic than during a stay on a regular ward. The reason for this is that patients in need of intensive care often are so affected from their illness and the drugs they are given, that they have problem to take part in conversation and decision making. Rattray, Johnston and Wildsmith (2004) found in their study that the patients after an intensive care stay experienced that they during the stay often did not even knew if it was day or night. Their memories were blurred and they wished they could remember more. But even under these circumstances a majority said they had known what they wanted and that they were satisfied with the care they had received. The statement that they felt safe but helpless, confirm how important it is that the intensive care nurse really take everything in consideration and acts like the intensive care patient's lawyer.

When a person is as ill as an intensive care patient usually is, it is of great importance to remember to cake good care of the belonging relatives and friends. They also undergo their potentially worst time of their life. Often they repeatedly need information about the patient's condition, prognosis and planned care. They need to be told about the purpose of all the things and machines in the room and what tasks all the people around the patient have. It is also important to give them time to ask questions and be listened to (Larsson & Rubertsson, 2005).

Gender perspective

Since men and women both work within the intensive care units and are in need of intensive care it is important to discuss whether sex makes a difference in the care. Gemzöe (2002) wrote that men and women often are described as each other's opposites and this makes it hard to show the natural characteristics that actually are like between the genders. Connell (2005) argued that the research within the sex difference, from the very beginning, has showed that there are none or a fairly small difference between males and females in all the investigated areas. This led to the conclusion that most personalities are individual and not female or male, why it is important for the personnel to interpret the signals from the intensive care patients right and try to understand how each intensive care patient would like to be cared for. The concept of gender is according to Magnusson (2002) about how women, compared to men, are treated by their surroundings. The most important point in the health care is to treat the patient as the unique individual he or she is. The question is whether that is done, or if the intensive care nurses tend to treat their intensive care patients as a stereotype man or women and less as an individual. To be able to find out about this it is necessary to identify what sex and gender is.

According to Nationalencyklopedin (2009:C) sex is the characteristics an individual have dependent on which kind of sex cell they produce. Compared to the word sex, gender has a wider and less strict definition. It is considered to be a social sex, developed from ideas and actions and it is also different in different cultures. Even if the sex definition decides about man or women the definition of gender can give both sexes male and female qualities (Karlsson-Minganti, 2007). Connell (1987) argued that gender is systematically organized and flowing through all aspects of human and social life. It can be seen in the thoughts, the actions, the dreams, the desires, the myths and in the understanding of one's own identity. In the society it influences on the categorizations, the work, the politics, the law, the institutions and the states. Even in the smallest families it is visible through the sexuality and reproduction and therefore also in the relationships to the relatives. Karlsson-Minganti developed this thought when she argued that each society has its own idea of how gender should influence on the chance to reach a particular social position or on how resources and possibilities of partaking should be distributed. One common issue of discussion is the order of gender where a general feature is a historic male dominance. Often the oldest man has authority in the family and men and women are referred to different places, roles and duties. Gemzöe (2002) wrote about how anthropologists have found patterns in all cultures pointing to the fact that men and women have been directed towards different tasks. A specific task has a male, a female or a neutral code. Whereas one culture considers a task masculine another culture perhaps considers the same task feminine. Each society teaches their children through upbringing how to act and how to be according to their sex and they are pushed into a stereotype role when it comes to behavior (Östlin, Danielsson, Diderichsen, Härenstam & Lindberg, 1996).

Jordan is now trying to make the society between men and women more on an equal footing. The United Nations international convention of women's rights has been signed, excluding the parts which conflicts with their national or Islamic laws. A national strategy for women has also been accepted and the Jordanian Department of Labour market has established a special department for women and their work (Heine, 2006). The Directorate of Women's Affairs has been established to safeguard the rights of women in the Jordanian Armed Forces and allow them to reach their full potential (The Hashemite Kingdom of Jordan, 2009).

Sex differences in health care

When a person is ill it is very important that the person get a chance to express oneself regarding the treatment and care when so is possible. Karlsson-Minganti (2007) found that even if a woman can imagine the possibility of free choices it is not sure she upholds this right if it is contrary to custom. According to Östlin et al. (1996) women may need the being ill role as a life role to confirm their femininity. Ancient customs tells the men the code of masculinity is strength and power and that physical weakness is more allowed for women who in general are ill more often but still live longer than men do. Often there is a socio cultural difference between males` and females` risk taking and tendency to seek health care.

Previous studies have shown that gender does have an impact on the relation between the physician and the patient. In general female physicians spend more time with their patients to give and receive more information, perform more preventive screening and talk about the psychosocial aspects (Bertakis & Azari, 2007). They also want to encourage the patient which can improve the health outcome (Bertakis & Azari; Stewart, Abbey, Shnek, Irvine & Grace, 2004). Male physicians instead spend a lot of time to take down the patient`s medical history, plan the treatment and discuss its effects. They focus more on the biomedical aspects and write more referrals for further medical examinations and invasive procedures (Bertakis & Azari). When it comes to nurses Kirchmeyer and Bullin (1997) found that nursing students often have a high feminine and a low masculine profile but when they get more experienced they tend to act more masculine.

Patients of different sex also tend to act different during the appointment with the physician. Female patients often ask more questions, send more emotional and positive statements and seem to be more involved in the care than their male counterparts. Male patients who see a male physician have the least participating meetings but they undergo more physical examination (Bertakis & Azari, 2007). Stewart et al. (2004) found that the younger and more educated the patient was, the more active he or she wanted to be during the appointments. All patients rated a personal discussion with their physician or nurse as the best way of receiving health information. Bertakis and Azari found that "...*good communication between physicians and patients is essential for quality healthcare.*" (p. 867). This was verified by Verdonk, Harting and Lagro-Janssen (2007) who argued that it leads to a higher patient satisfaction. Another interesting point is that patients in general expected more empathy from a female physician than from a male, which explains why they were more satisfied with a male physician who acted aggressive than with a female physician acting in the same way (Verdonk et al., 2007).

Sex differences in intensive care

Studies have found that men easier get enrolled to an intensive care unit and that women need to be more severe ill to get transferred there. Least chance to get a referral had young women (Arslanian-Engoren, 2001; Fowler et al., 2007; Raine, Goldfrad, Rowan & Black, 2002; Valentin, Jordan, Lang, Hiesmayr & Metnitz, 2003). Raine et al., Reinikainen, Niskanen, Uusaro and Roukonen (2005) and Valentin et al. found that even if women have a higher mortality rate than men there were no difference in outcome according to severity of illness. On the other hand, Fowler et al. argued that women died more frequently than men when they had the same severity of illness. Men also received a higher level of care at the intensive care units, for example they had more invasive procedures and received mechanical ventilation more often (Fowler et al.; Valentin et al.). This is a statement which has both positive and negative consequences because it could mean that it is less likely for women to get more advanced care, at the same time as advanced care sometimes means a higher risk of morbidity (Larsson & Rubertsson, 2005). Reinikainen et al. found that men stayed longer in the intensive care units but that they also had a higher postoperative mortality rate.

Kirchmeyer and Bullin (1997) found that nurses considered it important to have an equal mix between male and female qualities. It is worth noting that success in nursing, which by tradition is a female occupation, demanded a lot of masculine qualities. The intensive care nursing is a combination of caring which is seen as a female characteristic and technology which is seen as a male characteristic (Heskins, 1997).

RATIONALE OF THE PROBLEM

Jordan provides overall a good health care but the country consists of a mix of people from many different backgrounds. Often opinions about how gender related matters shall be handled differ between cultures and to be able to provide a qualitative care for everybody, a good communication with both patients and relatives are needed. That can also facilitate to achieve autonomy for the patient but it is important to be aware of the differences in gender that worldwide are seen in the health care work. The work in an intensive care unit is special and demands that the intensive care nurses use a lot of both traditionally male and female characteristics to be able to provide a successful care. It is also of great importance for the intensive care nurses to be aware of how they work since the patients in an intensive care unit often are unable to express their own needs and wants. This makes it especially exciting to explore whether male and female intensive care nurses work in the same way or if something in particular distinguish them. Since Jordan is struggling to make the conditions between males and females more equal, it is of immediate interest to explore if there is any difference between how male and female nurses, in intensive care units, perform their care depending on if the intensive care patient is male or female. To be able to do this in an adequate way it is important to understand the area of interest, why also the intensive care nurses presence as whole in the units was studied.

AIM

To illustrate how it is to work at an intensive care unit and to examine if intensive care nurses' or intensive care patients' sex influence on the performance?

METHOD

Choice of method

In this study, observation was chosen as method. Bowling (2002) described observation as a classic method to gather information within both sociological and psychological research areas. The reason for that is that it allows the researcher to systematic watch, listen and record the phenomenon of interest and in this way makes it possible to describe for example institutional routines in detail. Strongly settled routines have been shown to lead to a depersonalization of an individual in an institution and here can observations, if needed, develop into a powerful tool to promote a change.

> Observation of behaviors, actions, activities and interactions is a tool for understanding more than what people say about (complex) situations, and can help to understand these complex situations more fully. (Bowling, 2002, p. 358)

Observations can be participative or non-participative, structured or unstructured, quantitative or qualitative, overt or concealed and take place in a natural setting or in a laboratory. Ideally the researcher should observe an unfamiliar setting because it then is less likely that actions are ignored or taken for granted. Denscombe explains it as *"We tend to see what we are used to seeing."* (2007, p. 208). The choice to do a Minor Field Study in Jordan gave the possibility to perform the study in an unfamiliar setting, while it also wished to explore facts which could help the country towards a favorable change.

Bowling (2002) described ethnography as the study of behavior in a natural setting where the researcher tries to understand the symbolic world in the group of interest. These studies uses a triangulated approach which means data is collected in two different ways and analyzed separated from each other. When the two results then are put together and presented as a whole, each result complete and validate the accuracy of the other. To be able to catch both the verbal and non-verbal communication and behavior, observational studies often include both systematic observations, with structured information gathering through in advance created coding schemes as well as observations with unstructured field notes (Bowling; Denscombe, 2007). To give the result more reliability and make it more comprehensive this study has used both of these techniques. Denscombe explained that what brings these two different techniques together is that they both use direct observation which exclude what the observed say and instead focus on the behavior. They are also both carried out in the natural field and not in laboratories. This gives an opportunity to see things as they normally happen in their right context which adds a higher validity to the data. The third thing is that the researcher in both cases affects the result. The pre understanding can influence on how the researcher apprehends things and sometimes things perhaps are not what they first appear to be. To be able to understand and explain the observed activities it is therefore relevant to gather information about the background, why literature about Jordan and its culture was read before the study started. Conversations with people who live or have lived there as well as with people who have been there during studies or on vacation took place. These activities can according to Bowling contribute to reach a better validity since the researcher faster learns the social rules and norms.

Quantitative approach

In a quantitative observation study the observed object and the instrument for measuring are from the beginning specified and the study is carried out in order to test a theory (Bowling, 2002). An observation schedule minimize the risk of variations which could be a result of the researcher's own perceptions and emotions about the occurring events and it makes it easier to systematic and thoroughly record the data (Denscombe, 2007).

To collect and record data, an in advance created observation schedule was used. It contained numerous patient- or relative oriented activities, performed by the intensive care nurse in the intensive care patient's room. The observation schedule also included a part for total time in seconds, spent on the activities.

Qualitative approach

In a qualitative approach the observations are carried out first and out from them definitions and structures are found which in the end result in a pattern. Bowling (2002) explained that the content of the field notes needs to be restricted to what is observed and out from that they shall contain needed information about people, tasks, events, behavior and conversation.

The unstructured field notes were made in chronological order and caught whatever impressions the intensive care nurses and the intensive care units arouse.

Gain access

According to Bowling (2002) it can be problematic to gain access to a desired area for overt observations since people sometimes are suspicious towards academics and the purpose of the study. This makes it important to find a person who is acquainted with the area and who can help get an acceptance. Usually this takes time and often repeated communication with the head of the demanded area are necessary to be able to in official way give information about aim, method and value of the study and to assure confidentiality. In September 2008 the first attempt was made to get in touch with a professor mediated by the University of Borås. In October the desired professor at the University of Jordan in Amman gave an acceptance agreement to act as supervisor in field during the study. After that there was a frequent correspondence to discuss the stay, the study and its performance. To get access to the intensive care units during the study, the supervisor in field wrote official inquiries to the Jordan University Hospital in Amman. In beginning of March 2009 the hospital agreed to let the study take place, see Appendix 1. Bowling also wrote that it will contribute to a better result to let the future observed ones get used to the observer since that will limit the risk of people to change their behavior near to the observer during the study. Bowling and Denscombe (2007) argues it is important to spend time in the area of observation before the study is carried out why the researcher visited the intensive care units together with the nursing director's assistant in beginning of April. During this visit six out of seven supervisors for intensive care units were introduced and they all gave an additional face to face approval to accomplish the study at their unit. The visit also gave an opportunity to see all the units and be introduced to the intensive care nurses in charge for the day. Some shorter questions could be asked and answered and in this way the researcher was recognized once the study began.

Study criteria

Since it would give a more complete picture of the intensive care to see as many different areas as possible, four units were chosen for observation. The cardiac and the coronary intervention care units were excluded since they only have single rooms for the intensive care patients which makes it impossible to observe the events at the whole unit. The neurologic intensive care unit was excluded since it was not introduced as a possible unit for observation.

Twenty observations were conducted at the four chosen units, studying both male and female intensive care nurses who cared for both male and female intensive care patients. The observed intensive care nurse cared for an intensive care patient within good view from the corner of observation. Intensive care nurses whose intensive care patient was under admittance, prepared for transfer or out-of-unit-activity were excluded. Periods when resting hour or sleeping took place were excluded. Also periods of scheduled routines and change of shift were excluded since those periods are not representative for the observed intensive care nurse but for the routine care of the unit.

Description of the intensive care units

In all the chosen intensive care units the full-time intensive care nurses were working 48 hours a week on a three shift basis. Shift A from 7am-3pm, shift B from 2pm-9pm and shift C from 9pm-7am. Since the supervisors also were nurses and they had their rooms connected with the units they could take part in the bedside care if needed. Usually they work 7am-4pm Sunday to Thursday. The specialized practitioners changed shift at 3pm and the general practitioners at 4pm. The daily rounds were carried out 9am-10am and between that the physicians were either at the unit or available on phone. At the rounds the intensive care nurse in charge and the supervisor of the unit took part, more seldom the intensive care nurse responsible for the intensive care patient. Each intensive care patient was treated by a physician with the correct specialty for the patient's problem. When a patient with for example a medical problem was admitted to the medical intensive care unit it was not only the intensive care physicians treating the intensive care patient. Depending on the kind of problem, a physician with a specialty in for example infection diseases or nephrology was doing rounds every day. The specialist physician was also the first hand choice to give information to the relatives. All personnel cared for all intensive care patients, meaning there were no distinguishing between males and females. Repeatedly during the day cleaning personnel came to take care of the floor and empty the garbage bins but the intensive care nurses were responsible for cleaning around the intensive care patient. After a transfer the cleaners came extra to do a more thoroughly cleaning of the whole empty place.

Most of the documentation was done in paper case books which were kept at a table connected to each bed. Once every hour the figures were read and documented. The beds could be hidden from each other by draperies or movable walls when performing activities considered private. The intensive care patients wore long hospital robes and the females also wore something, for example a surgeon's hat, to cover their hair due to religious reasons. Clothing for the personnel at the hospital was uniforms of different kinds and colors. The students had special student uniforms or a coat covering their civilian clothes. Sometimes also physicians had civilian clothes under the coat. The females always wore long sleeves and some of them covered their hair.

In the pediatric intensive care unit (PICU) five intensive care patients could be admitted and treated in a big room and an additional intensive care patient in a separate room. Along one of the walls in the main room, a long office desk, the supply area, the medicine trolley and the utility room was situated, why the intensive care nurses never needed to leave the room while working. Three intensive care nurses worked on every shift. Filling up the missing material were the responsibility of the shift going on duty before they took over. Only the children's parents were welcome to visit and they could stay there whenever they wanted.

At the medical intensive care unit (MICU) four intensive care nurses were working on every shift and they had room for seven intensive care patients. Along one of the sides of the room the office desk was situated behind a wall of glass and beside it on one side was a place to mix medicine and on the other side the utility room and the storeroom. Relatives were welcome around the clock but were told to leave when special routines like change of shift and cleaning took place.

The first surgical intensive care unit (ICU) was more like a main intensive care unit treating as well surgical and medical cases and children before the intensive care patients could be transferred to the correct intensive care unit. The unit consisted of one big room with beds for eight intensive care patients. One corner was used for mixing medicine and storing equipment not in use. In an attached room supply was stored, in another was the office and just inside the entrance was the utility room. Four intensive care nurses were on duty around the clock. Relatives were welcome 8am-6pm.

The second surgical intensive care unit (SICU) could treat six intensive care patients at the same time. Five of them were treated in a big room and the sixth in a separate room, which in the first place was used as an emergency room. Along one of the sides of the main room the office was situated behind a wall of glass. Next to it was the storeroom and the utility room. Medicine was mixed at a trolley along one of the short sides of the room. The intensive care nurses were three on all shifts and relatives were welcome 1pm-6pm but no more than two at the same time.

Pilot study

According to Bowling (2002) it is impossible to achieve total objective observations but a pilot study can help the researcher to become aware of pre understandings and prejudices which will make it easier to stay objective during the study. It also gives an opportunity to get an overall feeling about the place, to find different strategies of staying as objective as possible and the first impressions from the unfamiliar setting can be thought through and handled before the study starts, which in the end leaves more focus to the observations. Especially when using an observation schedule it is important to make a pilot observation before the real observations start (Denscombe, 2007). Identification of which aspects are more suitable for quantitative or qualitative approaches can then be defined and shortcomings can be detected and avoided and the schedule is more appropriate when finally in use. The best place to sit during the observations can also be figured out, usually it is somewhere as unobtrusive as possible but with a good view over the whole observed area. To preserve the naturalness of the setting the behavior shall be as invisible as possible and preferable no interacting or engage in the work shall take place. The clothing shall be plain, preferable the same as the observed ones and jewelry and perfume shall be avoided or at least limited. It is good if the same style can be maintained during whole period of time when the observations take place (Waltz, Strickland & Lenz, 2005).

In this study a pilot observation was performed and evaluated according to Denscombe's *"Checklist for the use of observation schedules"* (2007, p. 216). It took place at the pediatric intensive care unit at Jordan University Hospital in beginning of April. The clothing consisted of a regular Swedish nursing uniform under which a long sleeve t-shirt was worn to cover the arms. The hair was tightly bound up but headscarf was not used. The observation spot had a good view over most of the room. During the observation as few movements and sounds as possible were made. The presence at the unit gave the intensive care nurses a chance to see what the study was all about and they could ask questions throughout the whole observation. This made them a little more used to the situation before they decided whether they wanted to take part or not.

The pilot study also worked as a test, whether it was possible to handle all the different methods of collecting data during the same observation or not. As a result the observation schedule was modified after the pilot observation and consisted after that of nine different activities. The activities noted were conversation with the patient, conversation with the relatives, have a look at the patient, have a look at the equipment, help with the patient's hygiene, administer drink/nutrition, give treatment, give medicine and training. For further explanation about the schedule's design see Appendix 2. Field notes were decided to be written down during the observation period instead of after since writing then became an ongoing activity and not only when the observed intensive care nurse carried out a patient oriented activity. It was also decided that each observation should be two hour long and take place either in the morning between 10am-12pm or in the afternoon between 3pm-5pm. The other time blocks were excluded due to the exclusion criteria. Bowling (2002) and Denscombe (2007) considered it important not only to include different time blocks but also different days to have a chance to represent the whole care. Therefore observations were decided to be carried out regardless off weekdays, weekends and holidays.

Accomplish the observations

Information about the study was, together with certificates from Sida and University of Borås, handed to the supervisor of each unit or to the intensive care nurse in charge before the observations took place. The study was also verbally introduced to the supervisors who then introduced the researcher to the intensive care nurses and showed round in the area to give an opportunity to get acquainted with the environment and find a good place to perform the observations. The observation spot was always chosen so that as much of the intensive care units as possible could be seen without being too much in the way and without observing intensive care nurses caring for the same intensive care patient during more observations. The supervisors of the units preferred to, on their own, introduce the study for the working intensive care nurses before each observation. According to the assistant of the nursing director no signed form of consent was needed. The supervisors at the units also did not think information to the intensive care patients or relatives was necessary but the intensive care nurses answered their questions if there were any.

The observations started the day after the pilot study and were carried out over the next three weeks to be able to cover all the days of a week. Altogether twenty observations were performed, five on each of the four chosen units. In the end both mornings and afternoons on every day of the week had been included at least once.

Ten observations were performed in the mornings and ten in the afternoons and five out of the twenty observations took place during the weekend. Doing like this, a better validity and reliability was reached since it was possible to avoid bias and get comprehensive data about how typical something was.

Since none of the intensive care nurses at the units disagreed to take part the every observed intensive care nurse was picked randomly to direct the observations so that five were carried out studying a male intensive care nurse caring for a male intensive care patient, five when a male intensive care nurse cared for a female intensive care patient, five when a female intensive care nurse cared for a male intensive care patient and five when a female intensive care nurse cared for a female intensive care patient.

Each observation started thanks to Waltz et al. (2005) and Denscombe (2007) with a ten minutes introduction at the scene. During this time the observer is supposed to act like during the study since the first ten minutes of an observation is the most critical ones; after that the participants usually have habituated to the presence of the observer. The longer time on site, the more the observer is taken for granted and the influence on the naturalness in the situation will shrink. The observations were after the ten introducing minutes carried out and each activity was noted in the observation schedule. The time was measured and written down on a blank piece of paper and after each completed observation the time was counted together and noted in the observation schedule as well as the total number of performed activities. The field notes were written down on a blank piece of paper. A new observation schedule was used for each observation.

Analyze collected data

The activities collected in the structured observations were counted together in number of activities of each kind that each intensive care nurse carried out around an intensive care patient or relative. From here the result from all the observations where a male intensive care nurse cared for a male intensive care patient, has been put together and is shown as a mean result of those five observations. The same procedure was performed with the data from the observations when a male intensive care nurse cared for a female intensive care patient, a female intensive care nurse cared for a male intensive care patient and when a female intensive care nurse cared for a female intensive care patient. The time each intensive care nurse has spent with the intensive care patient has then been counted together and in the same way as above a mean time spent around the intensive care patient and the relatives was calculated in each group. In that way it is possible to see which activities were more or less common in which group and how much time was spent on the relation to the intensive care patient their relatives in each group. The same procedure was used to count together the mean number of activities and mean spent time for the units. To make it even easier to read a total mean time spent per activity was counted and added to the above mentioned results. All the mean results were then rounded off to the nearest whole second or number of activities.

To analyze the field notes in a structured way Bowling (2002) recommended a method called thematic content analysis. It is a method that according to Waltz et al. (2005) can help find patterns or themes in a text. The systematic and objective reduction of the collected data makes it possible to divide it into smaller groups which can represent the whole amount of data. The performance in this study was that each field note for every observation was read through to make sure every sentence was understandable and did not need the surrounding sentences to be correctly interpreted. After that all the sentences which answered to the aim was marked with a highlighter. The field notes were once again read through to guarantee all the relevant sentences and not any irrelevant sentences were included. Then the chosen sentences were cut out and put into a pile with one sentence on each paper. The papers were mixed together and then read through and put into different groups in order to try to put sentences with the same meaning together. When all the sentences were sorted into a group they were again read through and, if needed, moved to another group which was more suitable. After doing this for the seventh time all the sentences were placed in a suitable group and fourteen different groups had developed. Now every group of sentences was copied to the computer to get a better survey. The groups that were alike were then put beside each other which created three major categories. All the sentences in the first group were then read through in order to find the common denominator for that very group. The found common denominator became the name of the group. This procedure was repeated for each group until every group had gotten its name. Out from these names the categories were named and a major theme which included all the categories was created.

Ethical considerations

Waltz et al. (2005) raised the question whether it was considered ethical to do observations in every area of life. Since this study was carried out in an intensive care unit it was likely that the observations would take place in very sensitive areas and situations. The decision to interrupt the observation and leave the area was therefore considered an alternative under constant reappraisal. For the same reason caring activities were not noted, only the time measured, while draperies were pulled to give privacy to the intensive care patient during a special procedure. Only once the researcher decided to leave the room, when cardiopulmonary resuscitation took place. It was after one of the observations had ended so it did not affect the actual study but it shortened the time for talking afterwards.

Under these circumstances it is also important to frequently remind the participants and the other persons in the area that it is totally voluntary to take part and that all information about single persons activities are treated confidential and nothing is going to be observed without the participants' agreement. To reach these goals the participants were informed about the study by their supervisor before it took place and they could at any time ask questions face to face or via e-mail about the study. Throughout the study information sheets were available through each unit's supervisor and through the researcher, see Appendix 3.

Health care personnel doing research are not only bound by the ethical principles within the human and social science research; they are also bound to their regular professional secrecy (Pilhammar Andersson, 1996). This was taken into consideration and also the role of being both nurse and researcher at the same time has been discussed. During this study the researcher acted as just a researcher since the Bachelor of Science in Nursing issued in Sweden was not valid in Jordan (Socialstyrelsen, 2008). However the attentions of the personnel were occasionally attracted if the intensive care patients clearly showed they needed help.

RESULT

Work within the intensive care area

The theme of the analyzed field notes is "Work within the intensive care area" which is divided into the three categories "Family", "Cooperation" and "Environment". To see all the sentences included in the thematic content analyze please see Appendix 4.

Table 1. Survey over theme, categories and groups from the thematic content analyze.

Theme	Category	Group
Work within the intensive care area	Family	Equality
		Solidarity
		Friendship
	Cooperation	Exchange
		Teamwork
		Education
		Trust
		Knowledge
	Environment	Crowded
		Patients
		Relatives
		Waiting
		Calm
		Silence

Family

In the category "Family" the groups are "Equality", "Solidarity" and "Friendship". It seems like the personnel at the hospital know each other well and that they like it at work. There is no visible hierarchy between different kinds of personnel, all have a function to fill and are respected for their profession and duties. Most of the time there is a mix of intensive care nurses on the shift according to sex and nursing experience. The big part of the personnel seems young and often it is livelier in the unit when both males and females are working together. They seem to get along well and they share both talk about work and everyday talk. The impression is that they act as a big family and that the work is more than just a work; it is a spirit of community which creates a good atmosphere.

Cooperation

The category "Cooperation" consists of the groups "Exchange", "Teamwork", "Education", "Trust" and "Knowledge". Cooperation between the units is common and equipment as well as medicine is often borrowed from each other. The cooperation within the units are also striking and many times it is difficult to see a clear line between who does which task since the cooperation are working across the borders of the professions. The intensive care nurses often work independent from the physicians but a task assigned to an intensive care nurse can be carried out by a physician, another intensive care nurse or a student under supervision; whoever has time and knowledge simply perform what needs to be done. There seems to be no prestige in knowledge but the intensive care nurses share information and give each other opinions and instructions when needed. It looks like there is a willingness to learn and experiences are shared. The intensive care nurses work close to each other and they have a good orientation about all the unit's intensive care patients even if they are responsible for the care of only a few. This gives opportunities for teamwork and to help each other out by caring for more intensive care patients if one of the intensive care nurses has a lot to do or if an acute situation appears. Also the education of the students is shared and the one nearest helps and explains even if another intensive care nurse is the responsible one.

Environment

In the category "Environment" the groups "Crowded", "Patients", "Relatives", "Waiting" "Calm" and "Silence" are found. Together they give the impression that it over time is very many persons in the rooms at the intensive care units. There is a mix of intensive care nurses, physicians, assistant nurses, intensive care patients, relatives, cleaners, students and people delivering or catching things. The personnel however seem comfortable with the noise, the rush and the limited areas. Even under high pressure the impression at the units are often calm and quiet and the most critical duties are spread and carried out without much talk. During calm periods, more frequently in the afternoon, the personnel seems understimulated and talk more to each other or take shorter breaks. Overall the intensive care nurses talk very little to intensive care patients and relatives. There seems to be poor information before different activities take place and most of the conversations take place when the intensive care patient needs to cooperate during a procedure. However, if the intensive care patient or relatives ask a question the intensive care nurses seems to listen closely and try to solve the problem.

Observations in time and activity

Table 2. Survey over all the observations performed with help from the observation schedule.

Observation	Unit	Nurse-patient (sex)	Time (s)	Activities (nr)	Time/activity (s/act)
1	PICU	Female-female	556	26	21
2	PICU	Male-male	551	21	26
3	PICU	Female-male	534	15	36
4	PICU	Female-female	504	14	36
5	PICU	Male-female	2388	25	96
6	SICU	Female-female	647	16	40
7	SICU	Male-female	1277	35	36
8	SICU	Male-female	1514	26	58
9	SICU	Female-female	1416	39	36
10	SICU	Male-male	3631	12	303
11	MICU	Male-male	1614	43	38
12	MICU	Female-male	840	9	93
13	MICU	Female-male	2101	33	64
14	MICU	Male-male	3340	28	119
15	MICU	Female-male	1359	17	80
16	ICU	Male-female	1408	25	56
17	ICU	Female-female	1020	19	54
18	ICU	Male-female	708	8	89
19	ICU	Female-male	532	14	38
20	ICU	Male-male	313	8	39

At the most 3631 seconds (1 hour and 31 seconds) was spent on bedside activities during an observation enduring two hours. The corresponding least time was 313 seconds (5 minutes and 13 seconds). Both times were measured while a male intensive care nurse cared for a male intensive care patient but the longest time at SICU and the shortest at ICU. The largest number of activities was carried out by a male intensive care nurse caring for a male intensive care patient at MICU and the smallest number while a male intensive care nurse were caring for either a male or female intensive care patient at ICU. The longest mean time to carry out an activity was measured when a male intensive care nurse cared for a male intensive care patient at SICU and the shortest mean time when a female intensive care nurse cared for a female intensive care patient at PICU.

Time distribution

Table 3. Survey over the mean figures for the groups.

Sex of nurse-patient	Mean time (s)	Mean number of activities	Mean time/activities (s/act)
Male-male	1892	22	84
Male-female	1259	24	53
Female-male	1073	18	61
Female-female	829	23	36

The measured time shows that a male intensive care nurse who cared for a male intensive care patient spend in mean 1892 seconds (31 minutes and 32 seconds) on bedside activities during a two hour long period while a female intensive care nurse who cared for a female intensive care patient spend 829 seconds (13 minutes and 49 seconds) on their bedside activities during the same time. It also shows that the number of activities performed were slightly the same except in the group were a female intensive care nurse cared for a male intensive care patient, in that group the number of activities were fewer. The male intensive care nurses who cared for male intensive care patients spent more than the double time on each activity compared to female intensive care nurses who cared for female intensive care patients.

Table 4. Survey over the mean figures for the units and the total mean figures.

Kind of unit	Mean time (s)	Mean number of activities	Mean time/activities (s/act)
PICU	907	20	45
SICU	1697	26	66
MICU	1851	26	71
ICU	796	15	54
Total	1313	22	61

The mean measured time from the units shows that the observed intensive care nurses at SICU and MICU spent more time bedside than their colleges at PICU and ICU. They also performed a larger number of activities and more time was spent on each activity. When the total time spent on the measured activities were counted together and divided with the number of performed observations, it occurred that in mean 1313 seconds were spent during one observation. That means 21 minutes and

53 seconds out of the two hours one observation endured, were spent on bedside activities. In mean 22 activities were performed during these two hours and in mean each activity lasted for 61 seconds.

Figure 1. Time distribution per group during two hours.

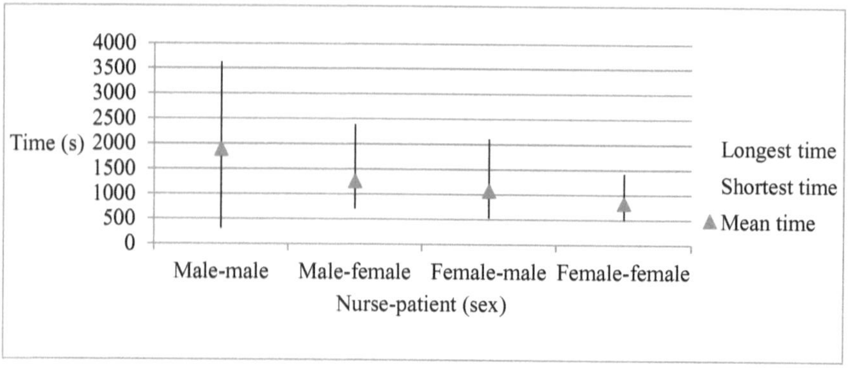

[Chart: Time (s), y-axis 0–4000; x-axis categories Male-male, Male-female, Female-male, Female-female (Nurse-patient (sex)); series: Longest time, Shortest time, ▲ Mean time]

The time span for each group and the mean time spent bedside during the observations shows that most differences in time are seen in the group where a male intensive care nurse cared for a male intensive care patient. That group had also the longest mean time while the group where a female intensive care nurse cared for a female intensive care patient had both the shortest time span and the shortest mean time.

Performed activities

Table 5. Total number of activities accomplished in each group.

Activities	Male-male	Male-female	Female-male	Female-female
Conversation with the patient	3	14	0	8
Conversation with the relatives	7	8	14	18
Have a look at the patient	27	32	22	19
Have a look at the equipment	50	32	41	44
Help with the patient's hygiene	2	5	1	2
Administer drink/nutrition	0	2	2	2
Give treatment	4	9	3	10
Give medicine	18	14	5	10
Training	1	3	0	1

In all the groups the most frequent performed activity was to have a look at the equipment followed by have a look at the patient. The male intensive care nurses who cared for male intensive care patients also gave a lot of medicine while when male intensive care nurses cared for female intensive care patients they also conversed many times with the intensive care patient and they had a look at the intensive care patient just as many times as they had a look at the equipment. When female intensive care nurses cared for an intensive care patient of either sex they conversed many times with the relatives.

Table 6. Total number of activities accomplished in each unit and total for the study.

Activities	PICU	SICU	MICU	ICU	Total
Conversation with the patient	1	22	2	0	25
Conversation with the relatives	8	15	18	6	47
Have a look at the patient	25	25	32	18	100
Have a look at the equipment	37	36	59	35	167
Help with the patient's hygiene	2	6	2	0	10
Administer drink/nutrition	2	1	2	1	6
Give treatment	4	12	5	5	26
Give medicine	20	9	10	8	47
Training	2	2	0	1	5

Jointly for all the units were that the large number of activities were concentrated on having a look at the equipment and secondly at the intensive care patient. At PICU also giving medicine was a frequently performed activity while at SICU the larger number was on conversation with the intensive care patient and at MICU conversation with the relatives. The least frequent performed activities in total were training and administer drink/nutrition even if conversation with the patient and help with the patient's hygiene scored low in some of the units.

In total it was possible to see that it differ some between the groups in how many and how frequent the activities were performed.

Figure 2. Survey over number of carried out activities in each group and unit.

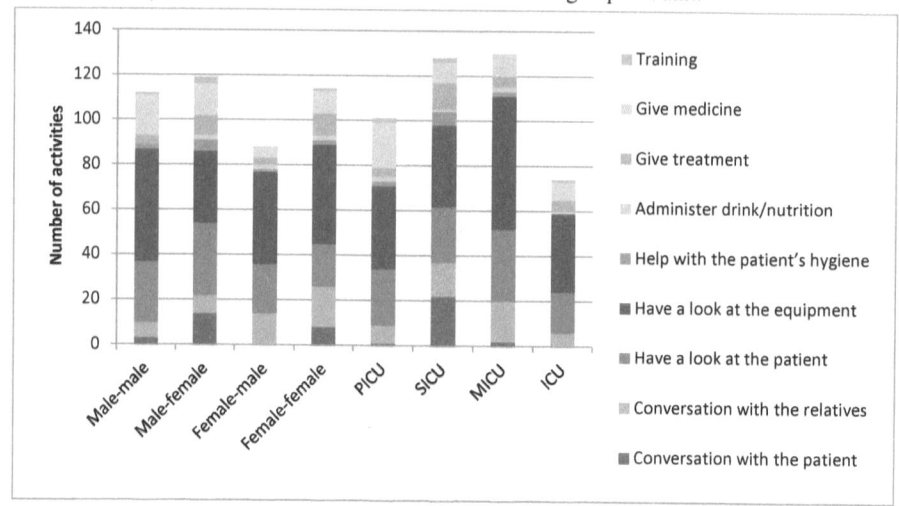

DISCUSSION

Discussion of the method

Since the researcher in this study was not familiar with the native language in Jordan, an interpreter or a translator would have been necessary if interviews or questionnaires were used to gather information instead of observations. That could have raised the risk of misunderstandings between the researcher and the participants (Waltz et al., 2005). The interviews or questionnaires could also have been accomplished in English but that would have been second language for all the people involved which also could have increased the risk of misunderstandings. The choice of using observation as method therefore appeared to be correct.

Observation schedule

The value of an observation schedule much depends on how appropriate the chosen categories are. It is important that the categories are carefully chosen since neither too few, too many or irrelevant ones will create good observations. Too few means that it will not be possible to catch all the features and too many means it will be difficult to have enough time to catch all activities (Denscombe, 2007). After performing all the observations the question whether the observed activities were suitable therefore has to be raised. Maybe it had been good to add some activities, for example preparation for/cleaning after procedure, documentation and education of student. All these activities were now measured within the existing groups of activities if they were carried out bedside but maybe had the result been clearer if they were their own activities.

Maybe it also would have been more correct to concentrate on one intensive care patient per observation, measuring time and activities spent bedside by all personnel and students. That could have given a more complete picture of how much time in total is spent around one intensive care patient and then count how much of this time and activities are carried out by a intensive care nurse of either sex.

It would also have been interesting to see how much time is spent on each activity. In this study it was not performed since there was no time to figure out a way to measure that in an adequate way considering different activities can be performed at the same time, for example medicine can be given while talking to the intensive care patient.

Field notes

According to Waltz et al. (2005) complementing field notes can be used to give a higher understanding to the structured observations since field notes are more flexible. They can enrich the collected data and help to interpret what the actions appear to mean to the intensive care nurse. This made sense because it gave opportunity to catch both the big and the more detailed picture from the intensive care area. The choice to carry out the study at more than one unit also contributed to a more complete impression of intensive care work. It is however important to keep in mind what Denscombe (2007) wrote; that systematic observation focuses on what is happening and not the intentions behind.

In the recollection of an observation Denscombe (2007), argued that the observer's competence and commitment make a great difference. He wrote that there are three things influencing how much of the observation that later will be possible to recall. The first thing is the selective recall where the memory is considered to consist of small pieces put together and every person remember and forget different pieces from an event. In the selective perception it is argued that some impressions are filtered away before it is even possibly to recognize them. The last thing is the accentuated perception which is depending on the emotional and physical state and the past experiences, which influence on how things appear to each individual. It is also of great importance to do the observations with an open mind, not letting the prejudice and pre understanding influence. The achieved orientation about Jordan facilitated the acclimatization to the new environment. Since all the impressions and differences from the past experience were put into print in the field notes they became identified and could easily be worked up and put aside before next observation. The fact that I am Swedish can however not be disregarded and the possibility that I found or did not found sex differences in the intensive care, may have been of other result if I would have been from another culture or had another background.

The field notes were from start all in Swedish but soon they were instead written in English to be more accessible for the personnel. The intensive care nurses seemed to get more relaxed once they had the opportunity to see what all the notes were about and could read for them self. Their suspicions about that the study was carried out in order to find wrongs in their performance were then eliminated. To take focus from the actual field notes they were mixed with impressions and activities differing from past experience. Those notes were the most read and discussed while the true field notes or the observation schedule did not attract much attention. Denscombe (2007) declared that it is important to make the field notes as soon after the event as possible to be sure to catch all the impressions and thoughts before they are forgotten or difficult to recall in the right way. The decision to write field notes at the same time as the observation schedule, so that writing became a continuous carried out activity, proved therefore right. It also made it possible to observe more hidden since the attention was not on one single person but on all the ongoing activities.

Access

Even if some things maybe benefitted by the chosen method other things were more problematic. Pilhammar Andersson (1996) argued that the behavior of the participants sometimes can be influenced by how the approval of the study has been handled. For example people can feel like being under investigation if the employer is the one who has introduced the researcher. In this study the approval from the nursing director and the introduction from her assistant meant no one of the supervisors for the units were questioning the presence of the researcher, at least not out loud. Despite that the supervisors informed the intensive care nurses about the aim of the study they were not convinced it was the true aim and rumors about other aims were going around. This sometimes affected the observations since the intensive care nurses then gave priority to other activities, for example infection control. The choice that the supervisors for each unit introduced the study to their intensive care nurses also left a lot of their questions unanswered why they later approached the researcher to ask them. This sometimes made it difficult to carry out the observations uninterrupted but at the same time it is not sure the observations would have been easier to carry out even if the researcher had given the information from the beginning.

Another thing Pilhammar Andersson (1996) found important to be aware of, is who the gatekeeper is; the one who decides when and where the study can take place. The risk is that the gatekeeper put up invisible obstacles forcing the researcher to see what the gatekeeper want to show. Throughout the study the researcher could, together with the supervisors for the units, plan when and where to perform the observations and not on one occasion the wishes were a result of compromising. What was surprising was the fact that there were seven and not six intensive care units at the hospital. This was revealed only after the study had started why the neurologic intensive care unit never was considered to be included.

Performance

Even if the study criteria excluded a wide range of possible observations many other influencing factors can still be found in the performed ones. The grade of sickness of the intensive care patient the observed intensive care nurse cared for ranged from stabile to critical, why the measurement of both time and number of activities may have been affected by this. The intensive care nurses were also always caring for at least one more intensive care patient why the amount of time needed for this/those intensive care patient/patients influenced on the time left for the measured care. The intensive care patients and their relatives at the units also had individual demands and expectations on the care why they in different degrees called upon attention, making the intensive care nurse spend more or less time bedside. Sometimes also relatives, students, physicians or other intensive care nurses performed care the observed intensive care nurse most possible should have done, if no one else had. It is also possible the intensive care nurses as a group or by personal causes, partly avoided to care bedside since they knew an observation study on what they did, was carried out. The subject of the daily mood for each intensive care nurse can also have been a reason for the care being able to observe. It is also possible that the intensive care nurses were acting different the first time an observation took place compared to when they had been participating in some observations, since they then maybe felt more comfortable in the situation.

Denscombe's (2007) and Waltz et al's. (2005) idea of coming a little earlier than necessary to the unit to let the intensive care nurses get used to the presence, worked time to time. Especially well it worked in the afternoons since the intensive care nurses working on A-shift still were there and could introduce the circumstances of the study to the B-shift. It seemed like the intensive care nurses were more relaxed having heard about the study from their own colleges and not only from the supervisor or the researcher. Even so, it was difficult to direct all the questions to before or after the observation since the intensive care nurses, as well as physicians, students, supervisors and relatives asked their questions when they had time, often during the observation. Sometimes that made it a real challenge to both observe and give a thought-out answer at the same time. This problem often increased with the time being at the unit. In the beginning the personnel were more distanced but after getting used to the situation, more and more questions were raised and the researcher was sometimes almost included in the personnel group. It was hard to find a good balance between being new at the unit when the personnel were suspicious and maybe not behaving as they normally would and being known at the unit which made the intensive care nurses work more easily but also more often start conversations.

Trying to avoid too much talk during the next observations the researcher tried to stay behind after the observations to do some talking, which to some point worked. These facts also point towards that it probably was wise to perform observations at different units and not only in one. However, since the personnel within the intensive care division seems to know each other well, the word about the study could have gone around to a unit before the observations took place. This could have influenced on the behavior on the later observed units.

Another act to decrease the interruption was to sit in the intensive care patients' room doing the observations and not at a spot in the office. In that way the researcher was more in the middle of things but the conversations were less since the intensive care nurses, if they had a few minutes to spare, sat down in the office. There seemed to be no difference in the reactions from the relatives in regard to the chosen place to sit.

Discussion of the result

Bierman (2007) argued that the most possible is that the patient, the provider and the system together create whatever gender differences there are in quality and outcome from intensive care. This statement emphasizes the fact that in an area like this, it is not likely to find just one reason for an event. Many things are working together to end up in a particular way and this study is not an exception. Bertakis and Azari wrote that *"It is important to keep in mind that gender is only one of many factors that influence physician-patient interaction"* (2007, p. 860). This can be an opinion to keep in mind even if their study focuses on physicians instead of intensive care nurses. Another important statement to take into consideration is the fact that males and females through their raising are implemented with different attitudes in how they should react according to their sex (Gemzöe, 2002; Magnusson, 2002). But we are all unique why all human beings can not just be sorted into a group of either man or woman. Therefore the only thing that actually can be observed in a study like this is the behavior of an individual and from that it might be possible to tell if men or women in general tend to spend more time on a specific activity or if there is no visible connection to the sex. Magnusson (2002) wrote about this phenomenon when she described that there are often bigger differences between women or men in a group than the mean difference between the two groups. In 2007 Verdonk et al. published an article illustrating the fact that the common medical education does not generate equal attitudes between the genders when it comes to what the students expect from each other, depending on the sex, in their profession. Even if the observation schedule in this study showed some differences in the behavior, no field notes in particular pointed towards sex differences in the care.

Communication

Fowler et al. (2007) wrote that men are often transferred to intensive care units after elective surgery while women more often suffer from a medical illness and are transferred from an emergency clinic or a ward. The males are therefore maybe better prepared since they could have gotten information before the surgery about the possibility to afterwards need to stay at an intensive care unit for a while. If so, these male intensive care patients maybe require less information during the stay, which would explain the few times conversation took place between the intensive care nurses and the male intensive care patients compared to the female intensive care patients. Another possibility, which would support Bertakis and Azari's (2007) research about physician-patient interaction, is that a female patient wants to be more involved in the care and asks more questions compared to a male patient.

The common view is that a relative, by visiting a lot, shows that he or she are concerned and cares for the patient. That is one reason to why relatives were around, sometimes round the clock and many of them took in the meantime a big responsibility regarding the care. Often they helped or took care of hygiene, mobilization and adjusting clothes, bedclothes and attached equipment. They therefore see most of the care and become well informed about the situation. By passing this knowledge to next relative the need to talk to the intensive care nurses might shrink. The female intensive care nurses however talked more times to the relatives then the male intensive care nurses did. The only of Larsson and Rubertsson's (2005) factors to be able to provide a good intensive care that was not fulfilled, was the importance of conversation with patients and relatives to find out about the patient's wishes and the relatives' needs. This can according to Rattray et al. (2004) be of less importance since they argued the personnel in most situations, thanks to their experience, act in line with the patient's wishes.

Priority according to interest

Overall this study showed that a lot of the activities performed were concentrated on monitoring the equipment. Heskins (1997) explained that within areas where the patient is not able to talk, caring is sometimes considered being a low priority compared to looking after technology. Her interviews with intensive care nurses however showed that they thought there were no differences between male and female intensive care nurses when it came to caring. Instead they thought it depended more on the individual caring interest and they found caring being the most important activity in front of technology. The only group in this study who, by looking at the observation schedule, performed caring activities just as frequent as monitoring equipment was when a male intensive care nurse cared for a female intensive care patient. The difference here could depend on the males being nervous about missing something since a common opinion in Jordan is that a female nurse should care for a female patient.

The fact that the male intensive care nurses spend the longest times both bedside and per activity speak against Bertakis and Azari (2007) who argued that female physicians spend more time with the patients then their male counterparts. This study's result also raise the question whether the female intensive care nurses work more effective or if the males are more thoroughly. The male intensive care nurses' long times could however be pure coincidence since the males also spend the shortest time bedside. Another explanation to the males' longer times could be that the most frequent performed activity is to have a look at the equipment, which Bertakis and Azari argue is one of the tasks male physicians concentrate upon. Maybe this also applies to intensive care nurses. The reason to why this activity is the most frequent performed can maybe be explained by Kirchmeyer and Bullin (1997) opinion that the more experienced a nurse is the more masculine the behavior becomes.

The draperies were frequently used in the units to give privacy to the patients during special procedures. During these occasions the time was measured but the activities not noted why the number of performed activities probably is higher than what the result shows.

Severity in illness

The amount of performed activities were less when a female intensive care nurse cared for a male intensive care patient which raises the question whether the male intensive care patients are less severe ill than the females and maybe are admitted to the intensive care unit on easier premises. If so, it would support the findings of Arslanian-Engoren (2001), Fowler et al. (2007), Reinikainen et al. (2005) and Valentin et al. (2003) but partly speak against Raine et al. (2002). Raine et al. found that males easier were admitted for intensive care if suffering from myocardial infarction or neurological bleeding but that there were no gender difference in the conditions primary brain injury, pneumonia or ventricular failure. This study's result is also divided since if male intensive care patients would be admitted on easier premises, the activities should be few also when a male intensive care nurse cares for a male intensive care patient, which they were not. The fact can also mean that the intensive care nurses who spend long time bedside have no problem with being under observation or maybe they are nervous about it and that is why things take a long time to perform.

Differences in organization

The result could be deceptive since both the physicians and the supervisors are involved in the treatment and close care and are helping when there is much to do. Also the students perform a lot of the care on their own, of course under supervision but most of them were last year bachelor or master students, which mean they have come far in their education. Therefore they were capable of performing most of the care, if not with help from an intensive care nurse, there were physicians, other students or teachers from the university there to guide them. The high scores of time and activities in SICU and MICU raise the question whether they provide a more advanced and demanding care than PICU and ICU. It could also be that PICU and ICU let students perform more tasks or that they have another way to work which facilitate for the intensive care nurses to care more for the intensive care patients they are not responsible for.

Bertakis and Azari (2007) found in their study that female patients were more likely to be admitted to female physicians than male patients. A pattern like this could yet not be revealed during the observations between intensive care nurses and intensive care patients.

Quantity or quality

It should be taken into consideration that the observations were performed during calm periods in the days when no routine care took place why it can be assumed that the bedside time and the performed activities probably are both longer and more numerous during other periods of the day. Another thought is if more time bedside means better or worse quality of the care. A lot of bedside time can mean more attention is given, the care is carried out more meticulous and the intensive care patient feel more acknowledged. It can also mean the intensive care patient has no private time to rest and relax and maybe the intensive care nurses are caring to much and by that harming more than helping.

Practical implications

The good spirit in the units are important to keep; happy personnel that like what they are working with will probably give a more personal and careful care. A part of this is to continue the work with mixed teams in the units, to promote and encourage the male and female intensive care nurses already excisting cooperation and support for each other. That will probably also result in the most optimum care possible for the intensive care patients. To be able to provide an even better intensive care this study suggests that it would be wise to include the intensive care patients and their relatives more in the discussions about the planned care and what is happening. It is also important to try to lower the amount and intensity of alarms to create a more peaceful and restful environment.

CONCLUSION

This study has in various ways illustrated things that can be applicable in the work as a nurse in an intensive care unit. The atmosphere in the unit in many ways influence on the impression as whole and talking to intensive care patients and their relatives is essential to not send out a nonchalant attitude. Much time is spent bedside even during the calmer periods of the day and even if male and female intensive care nurses seem to work different it cannot be excluded that the differences are more related to the individual than to the sex.

ACKNOWLEDGEMENTS

I would like to direct a warm thank you to the University of Jordan, their devoted Faculty of Nursing and especially to Dr. Halabi who has acted as my supervisor in field and answered all my questions. Jordan University Hospital and their wonderful staff also deserve a warm thank you for their welcoming attitude and fully cooperation. A warm thank you also goes to University of Borås whose helpful staff has supported me throughout my studies. A special thank you will also go to Sida for giving this opportunity and support through their scholarship. At last I want to direct a warm thank you to all my new acquaintances who has made my time abroad truly memorable and to my family and all my friends who have stood by my side.

REFERENCES

Arslanian-Engoren, C. (2001). Gender and age differences in nurses' triage decisions using vignette patients. *Nursing Research, 50(1)*, 61-66.

Bertakis, K. D., & Azari, R. (2007). Patient gender and physician practice style. *Journal of Women's Health, 16(6)*, 859-868.

Bierman, A. S. (2007). Sex matters: Gender disparities in quality and outcomes. *Canadian Medical Association Journal, 177(12)*, 1520-1521.

Bowling, A. (2002). *Research methods in health: Investigating health and health services* (2nd ed.). Buckingham: Open University Press.

Connell, R. W. (1987). *Gender and power: Society, the person and sexual politics*. Stanford: Stanford University Press.

Connell, R. W. (2005). *Masculinities* (2nd ed.). Berkeley: University of California Press.

Denscombe, M. (2007). *Good research guide: For small-scale research projects* (3rd ed.). Maidenhead: Open University Press.

Department of Statistics, 2007. http://www.dos.gov.jo/jorfig/2007/jor_f_e.htm (Downloaded 2009-05-28).

Department of Statistics, 2008. http://www.dos.gov.jo/sdb_pop/sdb_pop_e/inde_o.htm (Downloaded 2009-05-28).

Department of Statistics, 2009. http://www.dos.gov.jo/dos_home_e/main/index.htm (Downloaded 2009-05-28).

Fisher, W. B. (1996). Jordan. In *Regional surveys of the world: The Middle East and North Africa 1996* (42nd ed., pp. 589-630). London: Europa Publications.

Fowler, R. A., Sabur, N., Li, P., Juurlink, D. N., Pinto, R., Hladunewich, M. A., et al. (2007). Sex- and age-based differences in the delivery and outcomes of critical care. *Canadian Medical Association Journal, 177(12)*, 1513-1519.

Gemzöe, L. (2002). *Feminism*. Stockholm: Bilda Förlag.

Heine, S. (2006). *Två sorters drömmar: Kvinnoliv i Mellanöstern*. Malmö: Damm Förlag.

Heskins, F. M. (1997). Exploring dichotomies of caring, gender and technology in intensive care nursing: A qualitative approach. *Intensive and Critical Care Nursing, 13(2)*, 65-71.

International Press Institute, 2007. http://www.freemedia.at/cms/ipi/freedom_detail.html?country=/KW0001/KW0004/KW0095/&year=2007 (Downloaded 2008-05-28).

Jordan, 2009:A. http://www.jordan.gov.jo/wps/portal/!ut/p/c5/04_SB8K8xLLM9M SSzPy8xBz9CP0os3gDCyNfXxd3J18LazNjN3dPD2cDKNAPB-nAVGFqDFcBk ccBHA30_TZyc1P1g1Pz9Auys9McHRUVAceA2s4!/dl3/d3/L2dJQSEvUUt3QS9Z QnZ3LzZfMDgyTU1ER0JNODA2M0ZHSTUzMDAwMDAwMDA!/?WCM_ GLOBAL_CONTEXT=/wps/wcm/connect/gov/eGov/Home/About+Jordan/ (Downloaded 2009-05-28).

Jordan, 2009:B. http://www.jordan.gov.jo/wps/portal/!ut/p/c5/04_SB8K8xLLM9M SSzPy8xBz9CP0os3gDCyNfXxd3J18LazNjN3dPD2cDKNAPB- nAVGFqDFcBk ccBHA30_TZyc1P1g1Pz9Auys9McHRUVAceA2s4!/dl3/d3/L2dJQSEvUUt3QS9ZQ nZ3LzZfMDgyTU1ER0JNODA2M0ZHSTUzMDAwMDAwMDA!/?WWCM_GLO BAL_CONTEXT=/wps/wcm/connect/gov/eGov/Home/About+Jordan/Government (Downloaded 2009-05-28).

Karlsson Minganti, P. (2007). *Muslima: Islamisk väckelse och unga muslimska kvinnors förhandlingar om genus i det samtida Sverige*. Stockholm: Carlsson Bokförlag.

King Abdullah II, 2008. http://www.kingabdullah.jo/main.php?main_page =0&lang_hm ka1=1 (Downloaded 2009-05-28).

Kirchmeyer, C., & Bullin, C. (1997). Gender roles in a traditionally female occupation: A study of emergency, operating, intensive care and psychiatric nurses. *Journal of Vocational Behavior, 50*, 78-95.

Landguiden, 2009. http://www.landguiden.se/pubCountryText.asp?country_id=74& subject_id=0 (Downloaded 2009-02-22).

Larsson, A., & Rubertsson, S. (Eds.). (2005). *Intensivvård*. Stockholm: Liber.

Magnusson, E. (2002). *Psykologi och kön: Från könsskillnader till genusperspektiv*. Stockholm: Natur och Kultur.

Medicine Net, 2009. http://www.medterms.com/script/main/art.asp?articlekey= 24812 (Downloaded 2009-05-28).

Nationalencyklopedin, 2009:A. http://ne.se.lib.costello.pub.hb.se/lang/jordanien/ 217142 /217123 (Downloaded 2009-05-28).

Nationalencyklopedin, 2009:B. http://ne.se.lib.costello.pub.hb.se/lang/jordanien/ 217142/217125 (Downloaded 2009-05-28).

Nationalencyklopedin, 2009:C. http://ne.se.lib.costello.pub.hb.se/lang/k%C3%B6n (Downloaded 2009-05-31).

Pilhammar Andersson, E. (1996). *Etnografi i det vårdpedagogiska fältet: En jakt efter ledtrådar*. Lund: Studentlitteratur.

Programkontoret, 2009. http://www.programkontoret.se/Global/program/athena/ Mojliga _samarbetslander_prog._Athena-MFS-LP_2009.pdf (Downloaded 2009-05-27).

Raine, R., Goldfrad, C., Rowan, K., & Black, N. (2002). Influence of patient gender on admission to intensive care. *Journal of Epidemiology and Community Health, 56(6)*, 418-423.

Rattray, J., Johnston, M., & Wildsmith, J. A. W. (2004). The intensive care experience: Development of the ICE questionnaire. *Journal of Advanced Nursing, 47(1)*, 64-73.

Reinikainen, M., Niskanen, M., Uusaro, A., & Roukonen, E. (2005). Impact of gender on treatment and outcome of ICU patients. *Acta Anaesthesiologica Scandinavica, 49*, 984-990.

Sida, 2008. http://www.sida.se/sida/jsp/sida.jsp?d=115&a=709&language=en_US (Downloaded 2009-05-27).

Sida, 2009. http://www.sida.se/sida/jsp/sida.jsp?d=1747&a=1012&language=en_US (Downloaded 2009-05-27).

Socialstyrelsen, 2008. http://www.socialstyrelsen.se/Amnesord/utbildning_o_kompetens/legitimationer/Intygforerkannande.htm (Downloaded 2009-05-31).

Stewart, D. E., Abbey, S. E., Shnek, Z. M., Irvine, J., & Grace, S. L. (2004). Gender differences in health information needs and decisional preferences in patients recovering from an acute ischemic coronary event. *Psychosomatic Medicine, 66*, 42–48.

The Hashemite Kingdom of Jordan, 2009. http://www.kinghussein.gov.jo/government5.html (Downloaded 2009-05-28).

UJ Hospital, 2006. http://www.ju.edu.jo/medical/hospital/pages/medicalservices.aspx (Downloaded 2009-05-29).

UJ Hospital, 2009. http://www.ju.edu.jo/medical/hospital/pages/aboutus.aspx (Downloaded 2009-05-29).

Valentin, A., Jordan, B., Lang, T., Hiesmayr, M., & Metnitz, P. G. H. (2003). Gender-related differences in intensive care: A multiple-center cohort study of therapeutic interventions and outcome in critically ill patients. *Critical Care Medicine, 31(7)*, 1901-1907.

Verdonk, P., Harting, A. J., & Lagro-Janssen, T. L. M. (2007). Does equal education generate equal attitudes?: Gender differences in medical students` attitudes toward the ideal physician. *Teaching and Learning in Medicine, 19(1)*, 9-13.

Waltz, C. F., Strickland, O. L., & Lenz, E. R. (2005). *Measurement in nursing and health research* (3rd ed.). New York: Springer Publishing Company.

Östlin, P., Danielsson, M., Diderichsen, F., Härenstam, A., & Lindberg, G. (Eds.). (1996). *Kön och ohälsa: En antologi om könsskillnader ur ett folkhälsoperspektiv*. Lund: Studentlitteratur.

Appendix 1

Agreement in English from Jordan University Hospital

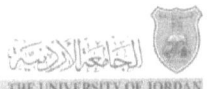

THE UNIVERSITY OF JORDAN

كـليـة الـتـمـريض
Faculty of Nursing

Ref: 2/1/2 / 722
Date: 14/05/09

To Whom It My Concern

This letter certifies that, "Katrine Alexandersson"; a master's student from the University of Boras, Sweden, has granted a permission to implement her minor project entitled **'The Significance of Gender in the Nursing in an Intensive Care Units in Jordan"**, at the Jordan University Hospital (JUH) through the collaboration with the Faculty of Nursing at the University of Jordan.

This includes permission to conduct research observations in the intensive care units at the JUH and according to the specified timetable during March-May, 2009. She has been supervised by the Assistant Dean for Development from the Faculty of Nursing.

Enclosed, please find the Arabic format of the formal approval from the hospital. For any further concern, please contact me at the address below.

Sincerely,

Dr. Inaam A. Khalaf, Ph. D. RN
Dean, Faculty of Nursing
University of Jordan
Amman-Jordan
E-mail: nurdean@ju.edu.jo
         khalafd@ju.edu.

Agreement in Arabic from Jordan University Hospital

مستشفى الجامعة الأردنية
Jordan University Hospital

الرقم: م ج/١١٣/
التاريخ: ٢٠٠٩/٢/

Ref:
Date: 2. FEB 2009

القائمة بأعمال عميد كلية التمريض / الجامعة الأردنية

تحية طيبة وبعد ،،

فأشير إلى كتابكم رقم ٢١٠/٢/١/٣/٨ تاريخ ٢٠٠٩/٢/١٥ والمتضمن طلبكم السماح لطالبة الماجستير من جامعة بورس تنفيذ مشروع مصغر في وحدة العناية المركزة.

لا مانع لدينا من ذلك .

وتفضلوا بقبول فائق الاحترام ،،،

نائب الرئيس لشؤون البحث العلمي والدراسات العليا والجودة
مدير عام مستشفى الجامعة الأردنية

الأستاذ الدكتور عبد الكريم القضاة

Tel. 5353444 Fax 5353388 - P.O.Box 13046 - Amman - Jordan

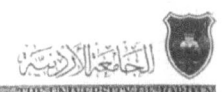

كلية التمريض
Faculty of Nursing

الرقم : ع١٠/١٢١٨/ ع.ن
التاريخ : ٢٠٠٩/٢/١٥م

الأستاذ الدكتور مدير مستشفى الجامعة

تحية طيبة، وبعد،،،

فأشـير إلى موافقتكـم الأولـية على السـماح لطالبـة الماجسـتير في جامعـة بوروس Katrine Alexandersson والتي ستقوم بزيارة لكلية التمريض في الفترة (٣/٣٠- ٢٠٠٩/٥/٢٤) حيث ستقوم بتنفيذ مشروع مصغر في وحدة العناية المركزة ضمن مشروع دراستها للحصول على الماجستير في الجامعة المذكورة .

أرفق طيه استمارة الطالبة Katrine Alexandersson الخاصة بدراستها المعنونة بـ -:

" The Significance of Gender in the Nursing in a Intensive Care Unite in Jordan"

راجية التكرم بالاطلاع عليها .

وتفضلوا بقبول فائق الاحترام والتقدير ،،،

القائـم بأعمال عميد كلية التمريض

د. إنعام خلف

نسخة /د. مساعد العميد لشؤون التطوير .

ع.ق

هاتف - ٥٣٥٥٠٠٠(٦)- ٩٦٢ فاكس - ٥٣٥٥٥١١(١)- ٩٦٢ عمان ١١٩٤٢ الأردن
Tel: (962-6) 5355000 Fax: (962-6) 5355511 Amman 11942 Jordan
E-mail: admin@ju.edu.jo

Appendix 2

Observation schedule

The observation schedule was created with help from Denscombe's *"Checklist for the use of observation schedules"* (2007, p. 216).

Activities/groups	Male nurse-male patient		Male nurse-female patient	
Period of time	10am-12am	3pm-5pm	10am-12am	3pm-5pm
Conversation with the patient				
Conversation with the relatives				
Have a look at the patient				
Have a look at the equipment				
Help with the patient's hygiene				
Administer drink/nutrition				
Give treatment				
Give medicine				
Training				
Activities/groups	Female nurse-male patient		Female nurse-female patient	
Period of time	10am-12am	3pm-5pm	10am-12am	3pm-5pm
Conversation with the patient				
Conversation with the relatives				
Have a look at the patient				
Have a look at the equipment				
Help with the patient's hygiene				
Administer drink/nutrition				
Give treatment				
Give medicine				
Training				
Total number of activities				
Total time spent on the activities				

Unit:………. Observation number:……
I = every time the intensive care nurse came in and performed an above mentioned activity

One of two different periods of time could be chosen for each observation, either in the morning or in the afternoon. One of the four groups' male nurse-male patient, male nurse-female patient, female nurse-male patient, female nurse-female patient were also chosen each time. When students cared for the intensive care patients it was not noted except if the intensive care nurse were at the intensive care patient's side giving continuous verbal or practical guidance to the student.

Elucidation of the activities

Conversation with the patient
Includes all talking and giving information about the present and following care and answering questions.

Conversation with the relatives
Includes all talking and giving information about the present and following care and answering questions.

Have a look at the patient
Includes inspection and observation of the patient, for example see if the equipment is correct attached to the patient.

Have a look at the equipment
Includes reading, changing and signing the adjustments and measurements, change, put in or take away equipment.

The patient's hygiene
Includes helping with washing, changing clothes and sheets, brushing the teeth.

Administer drink/nutrition
Includes giving oral food or drink, administer it through a stomach probe or start/end a nutrition infusion.

Give treatment
Includes changing bandage, administer or remove catheters, probes, tubes, drains and perform suction in the airways.

Give medicine
Includes giving oral, intra muscular, inhalated or intra venous medicine or fluids and start/end an infusion.

Training
Includes helping change position in the bed, movement training, manual lung training.

Appendix 3
Information letter to the nurses

Hello! My name is Katrine and I am a registered nurse studying intensive care at University of Borås in Sweden. Since many years back University of Borås and University of Jordan have practiced exchanges within the nursing division. As a result of this and a wish to see the life and intensive care performed in a foreign country I decided to try to get an opportunity to write my Master one year Thesis in Amman. Thanks to a scholarship called Minor Field Study, financed by Swedish International Development Cooperation Agency (Sida), I have been accepted to work on my thesis at the intensive care units in Jordan University Hospital between 30th of March to 24th of May 2009.

My intentions for the study are to explore what activities intensive care nurses perform for how long, during their daily duties at an intensive care unit. I am going to collect my data through approximately twenty observations in the patients' rooms. Only the voluntarily partaking nurses and not the other staff, patients or relatives who also are in the area will be included in my study. I hope to be able to perform five observations each in four of your intensive care units. Hopefully both male and female nurses in different ages and with varying experience of nursing will agree to take part, which will give a more complete picture of the intensive care. Each observation will last for two hours and during this time I will sit on a chair in a corner and note the caring activities into an observation schedule. To include the observation in the study the observed nurse has to care for a patient who is at the unit during the whole observation. To see if the schedule is relevant and to be able to modify it before I start my study I plan to perform a pilot observation at one of your units.

It is totally voluntarily to take part and everything will be treated anonymous. You can at any time and without reason withdraw your partaking if you change your mind. You can also at any time ask me to leave the room if you or anyone not included in the study would like so. When the study is finished I will make sure you will be able to take part of the result if you wish so.

You are at any time welcome to ask questions about my study if there is anything you are wondering about. For more information please do not hesitate to ask me when I am around or write me at katrine801@hotmail.com.

With hope of a giving cooperation!

Supervised by:
Anders Jonsson, RN and Senior Lecturer
School of Health Sciences, University of Borås, Borås, Sweden
anders.jonsson@hb.se, 0046 702 765619

Jehad Omar Halabi, Ph. D and Assistant Dean
Development Affairs Department of Clinical Nursing, University of Jordan, Amman, Jordan
j.halabi@ju.edu.jo, 00962 7 77762251

Appendix 4

Result of the thematic content analyze

The theme is Work within the intensive care area, including the categories Environment, Cooperation and Family.

Environment					
Crowded	Patients	Relatives	Waiting	Calm	Silence
Nurses, patients, relatives, assistant nurses, doctors, delivery people, cleaners	Does not talk a lot to the patient to explain the carried out activities	Relatives are around almost all the time but not much conversation with the nurses	Time for everyday talk	Very calm while cardio-pulmonary resuscitation takes place	Low sound level compared to how much is going on
All seems to like the pace, crowded areas and loud environment	Talks admonishing to the patient when not cooperating	Staff does not make speculations while relatives are in the room	Seems to be plenty of time	Calmer and more harmonious when only one sex is working	Quiet even if many patients
Overall very many people in the room	Little talk and explanations to the patients	Greet male visitors	No problem to take shorter breaks	Calmer in afternoon and evening	Without the alarms it would be peaceful
Chaotic because of so much staff	Patients can sometimes need more attention		Understimulated	Hard to see when the units is under pressure	Quiet shift, not much conversation
Less people in the afternoon	No talk to the patient to explain the procedure			Despite of stress the behavior is calm	No alarms, few phone calls
	Listening close to the patients´ requests			Calmer environment in the afternoon	
	Little information is given to the patient			After the round things calm down	
	Very little talk to the patient			Calm day	
				Calm	

Cooperation				
Exchange	Teamwork	Education	Trust	Knowledge
Units are borrowing things from each other	Hard to tell who is responsible, everybody cooperate well	The students talk to all staff, everybody educate	The nurses work very independent from the physicians	Continuous information sharing and learning within the group
Cooperation and borrowing between the units	All nurses seem to write in all journals and be by all patients	Students´ questions are considered and answered		Help each other with opinions regarding treatment
Cooperation between the units	One is responsible but everybody help each other	Students ask anybody for help when needed		All seems willing to learn new and are discussing
	Helping each other when a problem occur	Education of students		An openness to share experiences
	The nurse who has time do what needs to be done			Many shared speculations
	All the nurses seems to know all patients			Different areas of responsibility
	Acute situation, everybody are helping			
	Everybody cares for everybody (x2)			
	Help each other without prestige			
	Everybody help each other			
	Cooperation between the nurses			
	A lot of coordination			
	Good cooperation			
	Cover for each other			
	Overlaping work			

Family		
Equality	Solidarity	Friendship
No hierarchy or guarding ones territory	The staffs seems to feel happy, comes visiting after changed place of work	Laughter and work is mixed, serious when needed
Know each other well, like a big family	The staff tend to like the work, stay around to meet friends on free time	More lively when both sexes are working
Feels like everybody knows each other	Seems like the work, it is more than a work; it is a spirit of community	Higher atmosphere when calmer
The whole hospital as a big family		Nice atmosphere (x2)
All are a family regardless of rank		Good atmosphere
Everybody are a big family		Lively, cheerfull
Everybody talk to everybody		Touch is frequent
Familiar atmosphere		Much talk
No visible hierarchy		

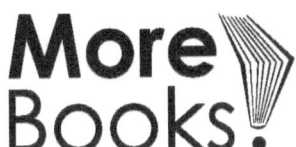

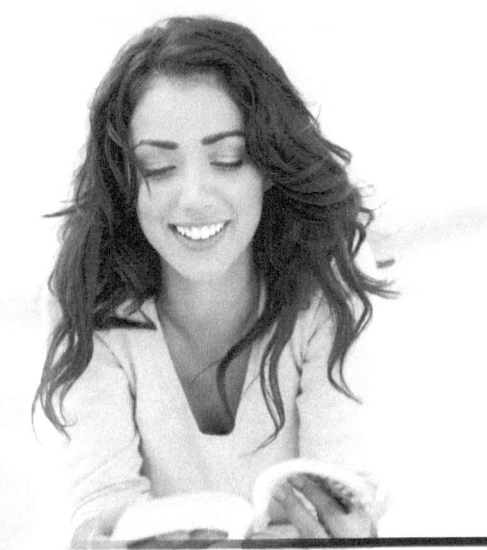

i want morebooks!

Buy your books fast and straightforward online - at one of the world's fastest growing online book stores! Environmentally sound due to Print-on-Demand technologies.

Buy your books online at

www.get-morebooks.com

Kaufen Sie Ihre Bücher schnell und unkompliziert online – auf einer der am schnellsten wachsenden Buchhandelsplattformen weltweit!
Dank Print-On-Demand umwelt- und ressourcenschonend produziert.

Bücher schneller online kaufen

www.morebooks.de

OmniScriptum Marketing DEU GmbH
Heinrich-Böcking-Str. 6-8
D - 66121 Saarbrücken
Telefax: +49 681 93 81 567-9

info@omniscriptum.de
www.omniscriptum.de

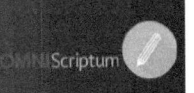

www.ingramcontent.com/pod-product-compliance
Lightning Source LLC
Chambersburg PA
CBHW031549210526
45464CB00003B/1214